Ketogenic Diet Rapid Weight Loss Guide:
Lose Up To 30 LBS. In 30 Days

Henry Brooke

Table of Contents

Take your results to the next level with these delicious Ketogenic Diet recipes books

Available Now On Amazon.com!

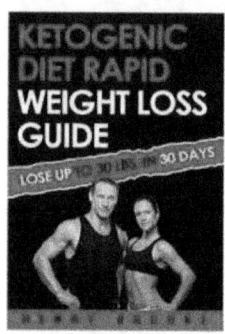

Ketogenic Diet Rapid Weight Loss Guide: Lose Up To 30 Lbs. In 30 Days

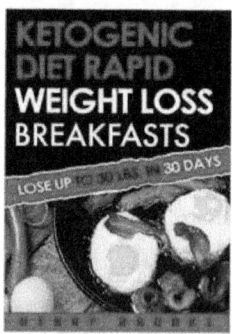

Ketogenic Diet Rapid Weight Loss Breakfasts: Volume 1

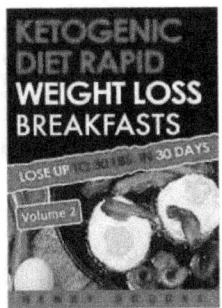

Ketogenic Diet Rapid Weight Loss Breakfasts: Volume 2

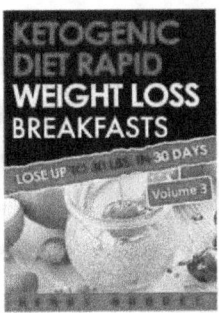

Ketogenic Diet Rapid Weight Loss Breakfasts: Volume 3

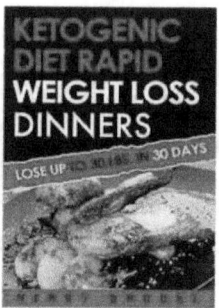

Ketogenic Diet Rapid Weight Loss Dinners: Volume 1

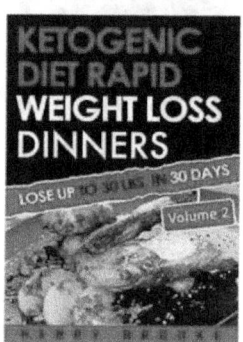

Ketogenic Diet Rapid Weight Loss Dinners: Volume 2

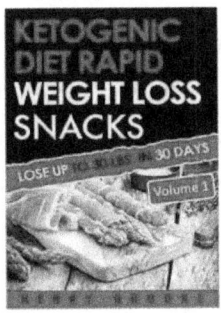

Ketogenic Diet Rapid Weight Loss Snacks: Volume 1

Introduction

Want to lose 30 pounds in 30 days?

YOU CAN with the metabolism boosting Ketogenic Diet Plan!

Crash dieting is something pretty much everyone on the planet has tried at one time or another.

NEWSFLASH - It doesn't work!

Livestrong experts report up to 65% of dieters return to their pre-dieting weight before the 3 year mark. That's according to *Gary Foster, Ph.D.*, Director of the Eating Disorder Program at the University of Pennsylvania.

The Ketogenic Diet can be used for successful rapid weight loss when used properly. And THOUSANDS of people report up to a pound a day lost!

This is an introductory take-action guide for understanding and using the Ketogenic Diet to lose weight fast and effectively. It will give you a huge advantage in forcing your body to lose fat and keep it off for life!

Nutrition and fitness professionals around the globe recommend healthy dietary changes and regular exercise to lose weight permanently. This is where the Ketogenic Diet comes in. An eating strategy that's not about starving yourself. It's a scientifically proven diet to lose weight that actually forces your body to chemically alter the fuel your body normally uses for energy. With the Ketogenic low-carb eating style you force your body to maximize fat burn for energy and blast fat stores in the process.

Is the Ketogenic Diet safe?

The American Journal of Clinical Nutrition points out no species could have survived millions of years without natural periods where glucose wasn't available for energy burn. Scientists also point out that natural ketogenesis occurs when you are sleeping.

And because of the high-fat intake the Ketogenic Diet allows calories to be cut drastically without feeling deprived and hungry.

There are thousands of people eating Ketogenic style that have claimed to lose between 20 and 30 pounds in just one month! *The Ketogenic Diet Resource* has success stories with people happily losing 30 pounds in 30 days and going strong!

We are going to have a look at the Ketogenic Diet for weight loss and other natural health benefits, while outlining a sample eating plan, food list, and exercise tips to help you reach your weight loss goals quickly. **FAST** weight loss is the focus and this eating strategy can make it happen for **YOU**.

This guide teaches you all about the Ketogenic Diet basics and how you can use this fast weight loss eating plan to rejig your body to use fat stores for energy first, while guiding you step by step towards a healthier lifestyle.

Don't miss out on this guide that teaches you how to take control of your fat TODAY!

Chapter One - Ketogenic Diet Overview

The Ketogenic Diet was created or developed in the 20th century to successfully treat young children suffering from epileptic seizures. It also shows promise with controlling weight and blood sugars in diabetics, and incredibly fast weight loss. I hope 30 pounds in 30 days works for you!

So how exactly does this diet work?

This Ketogenic Diet is an all-natural high-fat, moderate protein, low-carb diet that was initially created for medicinal purposes but has recently taken the world by storm because it triggers **FAST** weight loss.

In basic this diet switches things up by forcing the body to ditch the glucose usually used for energy and burn fat. Most people eat plenty of carbohydrates that are broken down into glucose and used for energy, particularly in brain and nervous system function.

When you systematically remove most of the carbohydrate foods from your diet the liver has no choice but to transform fat into fatty acids and ketone bodies. Now these ketones migrate into your brain for energy use instead of glucose. Looking at the medical end of it, a higher level of ketones in the blood reduces the frequency of seizures.

And for the rest of us, there's nothing wrong with burning fat, right?

Main Benefits of the Ketogenic Diet

Authoritynutrition.com recommends you have your blood work done before you start the Ketogenic Diet so you can measure your progress after you've been on the diet a few months.

Banishes Sugar Cravings - By having a solid healthy supply of nutrients in your system void of unhealthy simple sugars, your usual roller coaster of high and low energy levels will disappear, along with sugar cravings.

Decrease Hunger - *eatingacademy.com* reports ketone bodies take a big bite out of your appetite, and fat makes you feel full longer. Feeling satiated with healthy food is a HUGE benefit when losing weight.

Improved Digestion and Faster Healing - Carbohydrates are associated with inflammation, bloating, gas, and stomach pain. Removing them with Ketogenic eating reduces these annoying symptoms.

Levels Mood - Studies show ketone bodies help stabilize the nervous system which settles dopamine and serotonin levels and puts you in good spirits.

Increased Energy - Healthy protein and good fat provide great long-term clean energy. You will notice quality energy with this diet.

Weight Loss - For normal metabolic function the Ketogenic Diet is excellent for fast weight loss. Drastically reducing your carbohydrate intake reduces glucose availability and forces a chemical change where your body uses fat for energy instead of glucose. And by throwing in a routine exercise program you will intensify your results and look and feel like a million bucks!

Risks of Low-Carb, High-Protein Diet

Kidney Issues - If you have kidney problems you can strain your kidneys further by eating too much protein according to experts at *WebMD*. So check with your doctor before starting.

Future Osteoporosis - Studies show some people have a tendency to pee out more calcium than normal if eating lots of protein. This is something else to talk to your medical provider about.

Elevated Cholesterol/Increased Risk of Cardiovascular Disease - If you are eating unhealthy fatty meat protein in large quantities and full fat dairy in the extreme, you are at risk for increasing you cholesterol level and boosting your risk of heart disease. This is where you need to get smart about what you're eating and take into consideration your risk factors; lifestyle, goals, age, and genetic predisposition. Your doctor can help you with all of that.

HUGE MISCONCEPTION

You may have heard that ketosis is dangerous. You need to understand the difference between **Diabetic Ketoacidosis** and **Nutritional Ketosis.** Here's a little of the basics to help you understand. Your body produces three ketone bodies from fat and amino acids and manufactures ketones for survival.

FACT - Your brain only functions on glucose and ketones. And science says you can't store glucose for more than 24 hours, which means you'd die of hypoglycemia if you were forced to fast more than 24 hours and had no ketones. Luckily your liver can use amino acids and fat to make ketones to appease your brain's hunger.

Diabetic Ketoacidosis (DKA) is when a diabetic doesn't get enough insulin and literally goes into starvation mode. Sure they may have plenty of glucose available in their bloodstream but if they don't have the insulin to make it useable their cells and brain won't get it.

Naturally in defense the body makes ketones from fat. This would normally be a good thing but in a diabetic it isn't because there isn't a feedback loop to regulate this production or turn it off, and the body will just keep on making ketones from fat and amino acids for energy. Eventually this process will cause serious issues with the metabolic derangement of the patient and make them very ill. Ketones are essential but if they aren't regulated they will become toxic in diabetics.

This serious state is not possible in the average person even if they only produce small amounts of insulin. The feedback loop is created and the ketone production is regulated and safe. Yes it's safe to use **Nutritional Ketosis** (Ketogenic Diet) for fast weight loss. This is where the brain shifts and uses fat for energy instead of glucose, with the result of quick fat loss. A healthy individual losing fat with the Ketogenic Diet has no chance of experiencing DKA.

These two types of ketosis have about as much in common as a mud-puddle and the ocean. Now let's have a look at what you should and shouldn't be eating!

Chapter Two - Food List - The Okay - And The No-Kay

It's important to have the take-action information available to understand how to lose weight fast. So we're going to get down to business with an easy to follow food list for you to ensure you keep your pantry, fridge, and freezer stocked with Ketogenic Diet-friendly foods!

This diet is about eating **REAL** food. Look to stick with lean meat, eggs, yogurt, veggies, and sometimes fruit. Processed foods aren't on your list so steer clear of them!

GO FOR IT FOODS

Preferred Wild Free Range Animals Grass Fed (2-3 servings per day)

Pork - Ham, pork tenderloin, and pork chops (watch out for hidden sugars).
Whole Eggs - Free range is preferred and you can have them hard boil, fried, poached, scrambled, or deviled.
Fresh or Frozen Fish - Wild fish is best so you know it's free of any harmful chemicals or additives. Great choices are salmon, tuna, halibut, snapper, trout, and mackerel.
Meat - Grass fed is best and great options are beef, lamb, veal, goat, bison, and other game.
Shellfish - Lobster, shrimp, oysters, crab, squid, mussels, and scallops work.
Poultry - You want free range if possible and chicken, turkey, pheasant, and quail are great.
Peanut Butter - Natural nut butters are great. Be careful there aren't extra carbohydrates and sugar added.
Bacon/Sausage - Be very careful they don't contain fillers and aren't cured with sugar.

Good Healthy Fats (5-7 servings per day)

Note: Fats are a large part of the Ketogenic Diet and you want to make sure you get your Omega Fatty Acids by having 2-3 servings of fatty fish each week. If not, you should take a fish oil supplement just to be safe!

*Avocado, butter, ghee, and beef tallow
*Chicken fat, macadamia nuts, lard (non-hydrogenated), and mayonnaise
*Peanut butter, nut butter, and olive oil
*Coconut oil, red palm oil, and coconut butter

Veggies Minus The Starch (6-10 servings per day)

Note: Go for the low-carb green leafy veggies first. Choose higher carb options like shallots, carrots, snow peas, and green beans less often. You really can't knock yourself out of ketosis if you are choosing non-starch low-carb vegetables.

*Lettuce, spinach, chard, and chives
*Bok choy, bamboo shoots, celery, and radishes

*Seaweed, kale, mushrooms, cabbage, and avocado
*Avocado, okra, asparagus, fennel, and cucumbers
*Broccoli, cauliflower, peppers, Brussels sprouts, and squash
*Zucchini, tomatoes, artichokes, eggplant, and turnip
*Pumpkin, leeks, water chestnuts, and rutabagas

Dairy Foods (2-3 servings per day)

When possible full-fat and free-range are what you're looking for with the Ketogenic Diet.

*Full-fat whipping cream, sour cream, and cottage cheese
*Both hard and soft cheeses (feta, Swiss, cheddar, mozzarella, Monterey Jack, and Colby)
*Milk and yogurt

Seeds and Nuts (2-3 servings per day)

Note: Roasting nuts is best to remove any impurities and peanuts aren't really recommended, as they are a legume anyway.

*Macadamias, almonds, and walnuts are the best low-carb options.
*Pistachios and cashews are allowed in moderation because they are higher in carbs.

Note: Baking with nut and seed flours is okay in moderation.

Drinks

Your best choice is always water and you should be gulping at least 6-8 glasses per day. Clear soups also count along with herbal tea. Many people want to know if they can drink alcohol on this diet. The best answer is **NO** because they are loaded with sugars. However some people find balance with a lower carb option like vodka on occasion. Studies from *the ketogenicdiet.org* state people that tried to slip wine in ended up predominantly stalling weight loss efforts.

Moderation is key and if you happen to have a drink on the odd special occasion it's not going to kill you. Just don't make a habit of it.

No-Kay Foods on the Ketogenic Diet

Foods favored with this diet are typically high-fat, moderate protein, and low-carb. So a great example would be a spinach salad with grilled chicken, olives, avocado, tomatoes, peppers, Swiss cheese, and drizzled with coconut oil dressing. So it makes sense to avoid foods that are high-carb, low-fat. Make sure you aren't eating a giant plate of pasta for dinner or scarfing down muffins, pastries, or no-fat cookies for your snacks!

No Sugar or Diet Soda

You might think diet soda is okay for you because it doesn't have carbs or sugars. In theory yes, but experts at prevention.com remind us it's the artificial sweeteners that are the problem. Everyone reacts differently to them and the last thing you want is to work hard to lose weight quickly and have this oversight block your weight loss success.

Packaged, Shelf, and Processed Foods

Sweet and trans-fat loaded processed foods are filled with high carbs, and additives and preservatives that are nasty for your system. Processed, boxed, and packaged foods are usually full of sugar and all sorts of unhealthy ingredients you probably can't even pronounce.

Skip the fast food processed foods and opt for all-natural and wholesome when you're looking to lose weight **FAST** on the Ketogenic Diet.

Low-Carb Snacks and Sweets

Just because these treats are advertised low-carb doesn't mean they are. Many still contain processed food and lots of carbs. It all adds up so be careful.

Fruit

It's no secret fruits are full of carbohydrates. Which means you should avoid them for the most part. Even though fruits have natural sugars they are sugars nonetheless. In general try and stay away from high carb fruits like bananas, grapes, peaches, nectarines, strawberries, grapes, apricots, watermelon, strawberry, raspberries, cranberries, and blueberries. Find your balance and if you need to slip some berries in with your morning yogurt it's not the end of the world.

This includes fruit juices too.

Grains

These should be avoided completely. Breads, cakes, pastries, cookies, and foods made from flour shouldn't be on the menu. Breadcrumbs and rice should also be avoided.

Veggies Underground

Health experts from *Women's Day* report most vegetables that grow beneath the earth's surface have higher levels of carbs. Veggies like carrots, potatoes, and onions should be avoided when possible on the Ketogenic Diet.

Now that you've got the basics for what foods fit and don't fit so well with this fat burning eating strategy, let's move onto your sample meal plan.

Chapter Three - Sample Meal Plan

The first thing you need to do is figure out how many calories your body needs per day so you can set a plan in motion to reach your weight loss goals. If you starve your body it will systematically shut down to conserve energy. This means you'll lower your metabolism and your body will try and save the few calories you eat instead of burn more.

You've got to eat to lose weight!

You can get your doctor, fitness instructor, or nutritionist to help you with calculating the rate in which your body uses energy. Or you can just use a Daily Calorie Intake Calculator online. Where you use your weight, height, sex, age, and activity level to configure theoretically how many calories you are using each day. From there you can create your Ketogenic Diet weight loss plan to lose weight.

According to mydreamshape.com a 5'6" woman that weighs about 120 pounds that's 29 years old and exercises 3-5 times a week, needs about 2100 calories per day to maintain her weight. A 36 year-old man that's 5'9" tall and 175 pounds exercising 6 days a week, would need about 4400 calories per day to maintain his weight.

Having this number in your head is essential to lose weight.

We don't want to get too technical but you do need to remember it takes about 3500 calories to burn off a pound. The most successful weight loss comes from combining healthy eating and exercise.

VIP Pointer - Keep in mind you are looking to get about 60-70% of calories from fat, 20-35% from protein, and about 5% from carbohydrates with the Ketogenic Plan. For many people the transition with the carbohydrate reduction is tough. And one benefit of exercising hard is you may be able to push your carb intake up a touch and still get massive results without slipping out of fat-burning ketosis. Ever body is different and you will have to learn how well your body adapts to change.

Note: Don't be afraid to add an extra protein or high-fat snack if you are hungry. You may need more energy than a particular meal delivers.

*These meal plans are for the average women requiring about 2000 calories to maintain her weight. Add exercise to this plan and your weight loss will sky rocket!

BREAKFAST

Breakfast One

-2 scrambled eggs with 1/4 cup diced peppers, 1 tbsp. butter
-1 oz. slice ham
-1/4 avocado
-1 cup stir-fried spinach with 1 tbsp. coconut oil and 1/4 cup cherry tomatoes

Approximately 500 calories

Breakfast Two

-3 oz. smoked salmon
-1 large egg any style
-1 cup blackberries
-1 cup spinach pan fried in 1 tbsp. butter

Approximately 450 calories

Breakfast Three

-5 ounces ground beef mixed with spices, 1/4 cup chopped onion, 1/4 cup chopped peppers, fried in 2 tbsp. butter or coconut oil
-coffee with tablespoon heavy cream

Approximately 600 calories

Breakfast Four

Expresso Smoothie

-1 scoop vanilla protein powder
-Shot espresso
-1/2 cup full-fat yogurt
-1/2 ice-cubes
-Stevia to taste
-Blend

Approximately 300 calories

LUNCH

Lunch One

Grilled Chicken Spinach Salad

- -2 cups spinach
- -1 grilled chicken breast
- -2 slices bacon - chopped
- -1/2 cucumber chopped
- -2 tbsp. oil and vinegar dressing

Approximately 650 calories

Lunch Two

Cottage Cheese and Avocado Salad With Turkey

- -1 cup full-fat cottage cheese
- -1/2 avocado diced
- -2 cups Romaine lettuce with 1/2 sliced turkey, 1/4 cup sliced radishes, 1/4 cup mushrooms, 1/2 cup tomatoes, and 2 tbsp. full-fat salad dressing

Approximately 700 calories

Lunch Three

- -6 breaded chicken nuggets
- -1 cup broccoli pan fried with 2 tbsp. olive oil, and sprinkled with 1/4 cup cheese

Approximately 600 calories

Lunch Four

Ginger Beef and Spinach Salad

- -Slice 6 oz. sirloin beef grilled with olive oil and fresh herbs
- -2 cups spinach, 1/2 cherry tomatoes, 1/2 avocado diced, 1/2 cup celery, and 2 tbsp. full-fat dressing

Approximately 750 calories

DINNER

Dinner One

-1 5-6 oz. serving pan roasted salmon in 1-2 tbsp. butter
-1 cup mixed red, green, and yellow peppers cooked in 1 tbsp. extra virgin olive oil

Approximately 650 calories

Dinner Two

-6 oz. pork chop baked in 2 tbsp. garlic and olive oil
-2 cups shredded cabbage sautéed in 2 tbsp. butter and 1 tbsp. caraway seeds
-Side salad with 1 tbsp. high-fat, low-cab dressing

Approximately 850 calories

Dinner Three

Bun-Less Burger

-1 hamburger patty with slice of cheese served on 2 cup bed of spinach sautéed in 1 tbsp. coconut oil
-1 tbsp. mayo, tomato to garnish with tbsp. chopped basil

Approximately 600 calories

Dinner Four

-1 Mahi Mahi fillet sautéed in coconut oil and fresh basil
-1 cup mixed broccoli and asparagus topped with 1 tbsp. warm cream cheese
-1/4 cup hummus on the side

Approximately 600 calories

SNACKS

When you are in a pinch or just plain hungry here are a few snacks to keep your fat burning energy up! Each snack is 150-250 calories.

-1 cup veggies sticks with 2 tbsp. cream cheese or ranch dressing
-1 ounce hard cheese
-1/2 cup pepperoni slices
-1/4 cup almonds
-2 hardboiled eggs
-1 cup beef jerky (all-natural)

-1/2 cup chicken sautéed in tbsp. butter and wrapped in Romaine leaves
-4 small Buffalo wings (easy on sauce)
-1/2 bell pepper broiled and stuffed with 1/4 cup mushrooms and 1/4 cup cheese
-2 tbsp. almond butter rolled in Romaine leaf with 1/4 cup cucumber
-2 cheese strings

Don't be afraid to mix and match your meals up. Just make sure you've got plenty of good fat and lean protein in each meal, and easy on the carbs. Understand that ultimately calories are calories and regardless of which ones you choose, if you're eating more energy than your body is expending you aren't going to lose weight no matter what "diet" you are on.

I recommend you get some help finding your starting point or daily calorie burn from your doctor, nutritionist, or fitness training. This way you can create your own eating plan and figure out the best combination of Ketogenic eating and exercise to lose weight the fastest!

Chapter Four - Exercise Tips

The *Mayo Clinic* tells us exercise is essential for fast long-term weight loss, along with boosting your mood, lowering blood pressure, decreasing aches and pains, improving your sex life, and enhancing your quality of life.

Exercise also helps you...

*Lose weight
*Stabilize weight
*Prevent cardiovascular disease and stroke
*Ward off diabetes
*Increase energy
*Decrease sugary cravings
*Boost metabolism
*Increase motility and mobility
*Improve sleep quality
*Decrease risk of obesity

Need I say more? Exercise is a wise-owl move for everyone to lose weight and get healthy.

Here are a few exercise pointers to help you create the habit and make it worth your while!

Tip One - Start Slow

It's exciting to be on the Ketogenic Diet eating plan with weight melting off your frame. And when you throw exercise into the mix it's important to tame your bolt out of the starting gates. So many people overcommit to the gym initially. They plan to jolt their body and mind awake by intensely working out 6-7 days a week for an hour religiously.

What happens is you lose focus fast. It's just too much too soon. Experts say you are better to ease into training so it sticks. Start with a reasonable hour training session three days a week and work your way up. **TEACH** yourself to want to exercise because of how fantabulous it makes you feel and just as important how amazing you look.

Slow and steady wins the race.

Tip Two - Set Yourself Up For Success

Are you a morning person or a nighthawk? Do you have to get up ultra-early for work or find yourself completely exhausted when the 6 o'clock quit bell rings? You really need to consider when it's best time-wise to exercise.

If you know you aren't going to have the energy to hit the gym on the way home from work then make sure you plan your blast first thing in the morning. If you are the type of person that's going to roll over and hit the snooze button unless you've got a training partner meeting you at the gym, then find a training partner.

The more positive parameters you set up around your sensible exercise routine the better!

Tip Three - Do What You Enjoy

FitMD experts strongly suggest you find an exercise you enjoy if you want to make it a healthy part of your new routine for life. If you **HATE** being cooped up in the gym then maybe you should go for a bike ride, join a running group, or take up swimming.

Test out activities maybe you haven't tried before like dancing, playing soccer, skating, and even intense gardening counts. Just as long as you are physically exerting yourself for a prolonged period of time, 30 plus minutes of sweating, then you are on the right track.

Open your mind and start experimenting. Find the exercises you enjoy and get moving!

Tip Four - Make it Routine

Brainpickings.org suggests it takes approximately 66 days to transform a repeated action into habit. Which means you are going to have to program your head to "just do it" for just over two months before you can rest your head a little bit and not have to think so hard about exercising.

Beware that even though most experts suggest the 66 day mark to turn and action into habit, I think that's fairly lenient. I've read studies where habits aren't formed for 3-6 months, with regular check-ins afterward to ensure you don't slip backwards.

It's best to expect the effort to exercise will get easier after the 2-3 month mark, but some days you're really going to have to focus.

Tip Five - Use Cardio and Weight Lifting/Strength Training

Fitness gurus at bodybuilding.com recommend exercise programs should have both resistance training and cardiovascular exercise. Finding balance in building lean muscle mass to boost metabolism and blast fat while strengthening your heart, lungs, and internal systems, along with toning and smoothing out your look, is all key to a slimmer sexier you.

The proportion of cardio exercise versus the intensity of your weight or strength training is proportionate to your specific goals. If you are just looking to lose as much weight as fast as you can, it's best to build up your lean muscle mass with intense weight training 2-3 days a week and make sure you get at least 90 minutes weekly of good cardio.

You could walk moderately on the treadmill for 30 minutes and do 20 minutes of strength training pushups, crunches, squats, and lunges to start. Then repeat the cycle. Or maybe a 45 minute aerobics session is more to your liking. Where the instructor guides you through the cardio according to your conditioning level, and incorporates light weights and strength training moves throughout.

Whatever you do make sure you get both cardio and muscle building exercise into your routine!

Tip Six - Challenge Yourself!

This one seriously drives me nuts! If you are going to work out it's important to challenge yourself **EVERY TIME**! Have a nice Ketogenic style snack about an hour before, like a hard boiled with 1/4 of an avocado, or maybe 1/4 cup of almonds and a cheese string. Give your body some good fat and protein to give you the energy to build fat burning muscle and shrink your frame.

If you did 10 pushups last session go for 12 the next time. Maybe you were walking at a 5.5 pace on the treadmill your previous session, so kick it up to 5.7 next time round. And if you can't push yourself to work hard every session maybe you need to enlist in a trainer to maximize your workouts. Most gyms will give you the use of a trainer free for a couple sessions to get you started. That's worth serious consideration whether you are a newbie or an expert in fitness.

Tip Seven - Interval Training

HIIT or High Intensity Interval Training is the fastest and most effective route to lose fat, according to builtlean.com, and every other fitness expert in the world. HIIT involves alternating between bouts of high intensity cardiovascular training and lower intensity exercise. For example, you might run hard for a minute, then jog lightly for 5 minutes, and then pick up the pace for 4 more minutes. Many incorporate weight training in the same fashion as the cardio activity. What this does is trick your body into maximizing your calorie burn, keeps your mind busy and not bored, and consistently uses different muscles all the time, which means massive results faster.

So you could bike hard for 5 minutes, then moderately for 5, incorporate a sequence of pushups, sit-ups, lunges, and squats into the mix, and then hop back on the bike for another 3 minutes of really hard peddling. Then you repeat the sequence.

You may have heard having your heart rate consistently at 60-65% of your maximum heart rate is optimal for fat burning. That's crap. Provided you're fueling your body right, the higher your heart rate the more fat you are burning. With HIIT you can repeatedly push your maximum fat burn periodically to take advantage of the rate in which you burn fat.

Do you want to peddle at a steady rate on your bike for an hour to burn about 350 calories? Or would you rather change the intensity of your biking between bouts of hard, moderate, and moderately hard biking for 45 minutes to burn 400 calories?

Tip Eight - Shout it Out to the World!

Research studies show people that include the support of friends, family, doctors, and other influential people are more likely to stick with the program. You should be talking about your new Ketogenic Diet eating plan and exercise program so your social circle can help keep you on track to your goals. It's very important in the big picture of good health.

Tip Nine- Check In

Fitness experts from sharecare.com suggest tracking your exercise routine and results so you can measure progress. Seeing is believing! It really doesn't matter how you do this as long as you get it done. Some people might go by the way their clothes fit, others step on the scale once a week to check in, and maybe you want to focus with how you feel?

It really doesn't matter as long as you consciously pay attention to your progress once in a while. Just be sure you don't get obsessed with it as many do. Stepping on the scale every single morning is an unhealthy obsession, not a supporting factor in your healthy weight loss program.

Tip Ten - Journal

This may sound tedious by I swear by detailed journaling, particularly when you are just getting started making your eating and exercise changes. Start by writing down everything you are doing to get activity in your day. In time you will notice patterns and see the results for your efforts. This is very important in keeping you motivated and inspiring you to want more.

Actions = Results

You now have a tool to look back on when things aren't going so well and you can make the changes required to improve.

Tip Eleven - Keep it Diverse

Diversity is the key to life. If you get stuck in a rut of eating the exact same things every day and exercising the exact same routine you are going to get bored fast and your body is going to naturally become lazy and less efficient at burning fat.

Going through the motions is what's going to happen if you aren't diversifying your exercise routine enough to keep your brain and body working hard. You do **NOT** want to go on autopilot because your head is going to tell you that you should be making progress but your actions aren't going to add up. This creates frustration and often triggers people to throw in the towel.

Never do the exact same exercise routine and you won't ever have to worry about not getting results or hitting major plateaus with no results.

Tip Twelve - Accept You'll Slip and Fall - Get Back Up!

Life is going to throw curveballs at you from time to time that are going to send you off track. Accept this and commit to getting back on track fast. You may go on vacation for a week and slack off your routine training regimen for other fun in the sun activities. That's perfectly okay. Take this time to recharge your internal systems and get back to it when you are back to reality.

During the Christmas break you may be so full of family obligations that you miss most of your regular exercise sessions. Let it go and just get back into it when the festivities are done.

Tip Thirteen - Set CLEAR Goals

Many people fall of track with their exercise regimen because they don't set clear goals from the start. This may not seem very important but it certainly is. If you need a trainer to help you with this, use one. Write down your weight loss goals and time lines so you have a plan in fitness.

Be open to adjusting as you move towards your goals because predictions don't always turn out as planned. Just as long as you don't quit and you constantly remind yourself of both your short term and long term goals, you WILL reach them.

Tip Fourteen - Focus on the BIG Picture

Losing weight isn't about one particular component. You can switch up your usual eating pattern to drop a few pounds fast with the Ketogenic Diet, but if you don't incorporate the rest of your lifestyle to support these new healthy habits for life, you're going to fall off the track and gain the weight back again.

Psychology Today professionals say **BALANCE** is the key to a healthy lifestyle. You need to take care of your mind, body, and soul in order to find truth health. This means by committing to healthier fat blasting eating with the Ketogenic Diet, incorporating intense HIIT into your day, and making time for you and your social activities, you are creating a recipe for life long weigh loss success.

Always striving for balance in exercise and eating is critical.

30 Bonus Recipes

Breakfast recipes

Broccoli scramble

Serves: 1
Time: 10 minutes
Ingredients:
- ½ cup frozen broccoli, thawed
- 2 eggs, lightly whisked
- 1 teaspoon coconut oil, melted
- 1 tablespoon almond milk
- Freshly ground salt and pepper
- 2 tablespoons shredded cheddar cheese

Directions:
1. Heat oil in medium skillet over medium-high heat.
2. Add broccoli and cook for 2-3 minutes or until heated through. Combine eggs with milk until well whisked.
3. Pour over whisked eggs and season with salt and pepper.
4. Stir eggs until you have sort of lumps, for a minute.
5. Sprinkle over cheddar cheese and allow to melt.
6. Transfer to the plate and serve.

Nutrition Facts

Serving Size 167 g

Amount Per Serving

Calories 272	Calories from Fat 195

	% Daily Value*
Total Fat 21.7g	**33%**
Saturated Fat 12.8g	**64%**
Trans Fat 0.0g	
Cholesterol 342mg	**114%**
Sodium 228mg	**10%**
Potassium 315mg	**9%**
Total Carbohydrates 4.7g	**2%**
Dietary Fiber 1.5g	**6%**
Sugars 2.0g	
Protein 16.2g	

Vitamin A 17%	•	Vitamin C 68%
Calcium 17%	•	Iron 13%

Nutrition Grade B
* Based on a 2000 calorie diet

Frozen banana bars

Serves: 12 bars
Time: 15 minutes + inactive time
Ingredients:
- 1 cup almonds, chopped
- 1 cup cranberries, dried
- 1 teaspoon cinnamon
- ¼ teaspoon nutmeg
- ½ teaspoon grated orange zest
- 2 cups sliced bananas

Directions:
1. Place all ingredients in food processor and pulse until smooth.
2. Transfer to 8x8-inch baking dish lined with parchment paper.
3. Freeze for 3 hours or until firm.
4. Serve immediately.

Nutrition Facts

Serving Size 42 g

Amount Per Serving

Calories 74	Calories from Fat 37

% Daily Value*

Total Fat 4.1g	6%
Trans Fat 0.0g	
Cholesterol 0mg	0%
Sodium 0mg	0%
Potassium 164mg	5%
Total Carbohydrates 8.4g	3%
Dietary Fiber 2.1g	8%
Sugars 3.7g	
Protein 2.0g	

Vitamin A 1%	•	Vitamin C 8%
Calcium 3%	•	Iron 2%

Nutrition Grade A
* Based on a 2000 calorie diet

Breakfast fruit salad

Serves: 2
Time: 10 minutes + inactive time
Ingredients:

- 2 tablespoons pumpkin seeds
- 2 tablespoons chia seeds
- 1 cup almonds, raw, chopped
- 1 cup blueberries
- 1 cup thick coconut yogurt
- Juice and zest from 1 lemon
- 2 drops stevia
- 1 tablespoon coconut oil, melted

Preparation method:

1. In a small bowl combine coconut oil, stevia, lemon juice and thick coconut yogurt, until well combined.
2. In another bowl combine pumpkin seeds, chia seeds with lemon zest.
3. Fold in yogurt mixture and stir well.
4. Add chopped almonds and blueberries.
5. Gently stir and set aside for 1 hour so flavors nicely combine. Serve after

Nutrition Facts

Serving Size 206 g

Amount Per Serving

Calories 475	Calories from Fat 341
	% Daily Value*
Total Fat 37.9g	**58%**
Saturated Fat 13.6g	**68%**
Trans Fat 0.0g	
Cholesterol 0mg	**0%**
Sodium 2mg	**0%**
Potassium 460mg	**13%**
Total Carbohydrates 31.2g	**10%**
Dietary Fiber 9.4g	**38%**
Sugars 16.4g	
Protein 11.2g	

Vitamin A 0%	•	Vitamin C 38%
Calcium 13%	•	Iron 21%

Nutrition Grade B
* Based on a 2000 calorie diet

Apple pecan smoothie

Serves: 1
Time: 5 minutes
Ingredients:

- 1 cup almond milk
- 1 cup baby spinach
- 1 apple, sliced
- ½ avocado
- 2 plums
- 1 tablespoon pecans
- 1 teaspoon lemon zest

Directions:

1. Place pecan nuts and milk in food processor. Pulse until you have pecan nut milk.
2. Strain the milk and remove the pecans.
3. Pour milk back in the cleaned food processor and add rest of ingredients.
4. Pulse again until well combined.
5. Serve in a tall glass and additionally sprinkle with some pecan nuts.

Nutrition Facts

Serving Size 459 g

Amount Per Serving

Calories 137	Calories from Fat 31

	% Daily Value*
Total Fat 3.4g	**5%**
Trans Fat 0.0g	
Cholesterol 0mg	**0%**
Sodium 33mg	**1%**
Potassium 414mg	**12%**
Total Carbohydrates 27.9g	**9%**
Dietary Fiber 5.9g	**24%**
Sugars 19.4g	
Protein 2.7g	

Vitamin A 56%	•	Vitamin C 41%
Calcium 5%	•	Iron 10%

Nutrition Grade A
* Based on a 2000 calorie diet

Coconut-vanilla pancakes

Serving: 6

Ingredients:

- 2 eggs, room temperature
- ½ vanilla pod, seeds scraped
- ¼ cup coconut flour
- ½ teaspoon baking soda
- 1 cup coconut milk
- Small pinch of salt
- Some oil – for frying

Directions:

1. Whisk the eggs with milk, stevia and vanilla seeds.
2. In another bowl combine salt, flour and baking soda.
3. Combine mixtures and stir well until you have smooth batter.
4. Heat some oil in large non-stick skillet over medium-high heat.
5. Add 2 tablespoons, per pancake, and cook for 3 minutes and gently flip to other side.
6. Cook for 1 minute or so and transfer to the plate.
7. Serve with fresh raspberries.

Nutrition Facts

Serving Size 60 g

Amount Per Serving

Calories 136	Calories from Fat 106

	% Daily Value*
Total Fat 11.8g	**18%**
Saturated Fat 9.6g	**48%**
Trans Fat 0.0g	
Cholesterol 55mg	**18%**
Sodium 141mg	**6%**
Potassium 125mg	**4%**
Total Carbohydrates 5.3g	**2%**
Dietary Fiber 2.9g	**12%**
Sugars 1.8g	
Protein 3.8g	

Vitamin A 1%	•	Vitamin C 2%
Calcium 1%	•	Iron 9%

Nutrition Grade B-

* Based on a 2000 calorie diet

Ricotta breakfast parfait

Serves: 1
Time: 10 minutes
Ingredients:

- 2 oz. ricotta cheese
- ½ tablespoon lemon juice
- 2 drops stevia extract
- 3 tablespoons fresh strawberries, diced
- 1 tablespoon chopped hazelnuts
- 1 teaspoon lemon zest

Directions:

1. Combine ricotta cheese, lemon juice, lemon zest an stevia in food processor.
2. Pulse until all well combined.
3. Place 1/3 blackberries in the bottom of glass, top with ricotta cheese and again with strawberries. Top with ricotta cheese and sprinkle with chopped hazelnuts. Once again place strawberries and top with remaining ricotta cheese. Refrigerate for 20 minutes and serve.

Nutrition Facts

Serving Size 100 g

Amount Per Serving

Calories 119	Calories from Fat 67
	% Daily Value
Total Fat 7.5g	**12%**
Saturated Fat 3.1g	**15%**
Cholesterol 18mg	**6%**
Sodium 73mg	**3%**
Potassium 160mg	**5%**
Total Carbohydrates 6.3g	**2%**
Dietary Fiber 1.1g	**5%**
Sugars 2.0g	
Protein 7.4g	

Vitamin A 4%	•	Vitamin C 37%
Calcium 17%	•	Iron 3%

Nutrition Grade B
* Based on a 2000 calorie diet

Lunch recipes

String beans with sesame

Serves: 2
Time: 15 minutes
Ingredients:
- 2 cups string beans, cut into 2-inch pieces
- 2 garlic cloves, minced
- 2 tablespoon olive oil
- Freshly ground salt and pepper
- 1 tablespoon sesame seeds
- 2 dried chili peppers, sliced

Directions:
1. Blanche string beans in large pot of salted water for 3 minutes over medium-high.
2. Drain and set on kitchen towel to dry.
3. Heat 1 tablespoon of olive oil in large skillet.
4. Add drained spring beans and cook for 7-8 minutes. Set on kitchen towel to drain.
5. Heat remaining olive oil and add garlic, sesame and chili pepper. Cook for 30 seconds.
6. Add cooked beans and stir until well coated.
7. Transfer to the plate and serve.

Nutrition Facts

Serving Size 133 g

Amount Per Serving

Calories 186 — Calories from Fat 148

	% Daily Value*
Total Fat 16.4g	**25%**
Saturated Fat 2.3g	**12%**
Cholesterol 0mg	**0%**
Sodium 8mg	**0%**
Potassium 272mg	**8%**
Total Carbohydrates 10.2g	**3%**
Dietary Fiber 4.5g	**18%**
Sugars 1.8g	
Protein 3.0g	

Vitamin A 18%	•	Vitamin C 32%
Calcium 9%	•	Iron 10%

Nutrition Grade B+
* Based on a 2000 calorie diet

Veggie slow cooker goulas

Serves: 8
Time: 6 hours
Ingredients:
- 4 tomatoes, cut into wedges
- 3 garlic cloves, chopped
- 1 jalapeno pepper, diced
- ½ bunch parsley, chopped
- 1 tablespoon smoked paprika
- 2 onions, sliced into half moons
- 2 bay leaves
- 1 lb. green beans, trimmed and chopped into ½-inch pieces
- 1 cup corn
- 4 cups water
- 4 tablespoon vinegar
- 2 green bell peppers, chopped
- 2 red bell peppers, chopped
- Salt and pepper – to taste

Directions:
1. Place spices, water, veggies and vinegar in a slow cooker.
2. Cover and cook on low for 6 hours.
3. Serve while still hot.

Nutrition Facts

Serving Size 352 g

Amount Per Serving

Calories 79	Calories from Fat 6

	% Daily Value*
Total Fat 0.6g	1%
Trans Fat 0.0g	
Cholesterol 0mg	0%
Sodium 15mg	1%
Potassium 506mg	14%
Total Carbohydrates 17.2g	6%
Dietary Fiber 5.3g	21%
Sugars 6.8g	
Protein 3.2g	

Vitamin A 64%	•	Vitamin C 163%
Calcium 5%	•	Iron 10%

Nutrition Grade A
* Based on a 2000 calorie diet

Mushroom fritters

Serves: 4
Time: 15 minutes
Ingredients:

- 1 cup finely chopped mushrooms
- 1 small onion, finely chopped
- 4 green olives, chopped
- 1 egg, whisked
- 1 cup creamy cheese
- Freshly ground salt and pepper
- 2 tablespoons parmesan cheese
- 1 teaspoon dried basil
- Some olive oil

Directions:

1. Combine creamy cheese, egg, parmesan and dried basil in a large bowl, until smooth.
2. Add chopped mushrooms, pepperoni, olives and onion. Season with salt and pepper and stir well to combine.
3. Set in refrigerator for 30 minutes.
4. Meanwhile, heat oiled skillet over medium-high heat.
5. Scoop 4 patties, with ice cream scoop and place in heated skillet.
6. Cook until golden, for 5-7 minutes.
7. Transfer to the plate and serve.

Nutrition Facts

Serving Size 111 g

Amount Per Serving

Calories 187	Calories from Fat 137

	% Daily Value*
Total Fat 15.2g	**23%**
Saturated Fat 9.3g	**47%**
Trans Fat 0.0g	
Cholesterol 81mg	**27%**
Sodium 337mg	**14%**
Potassium 97mg	**3%**
Total Carbohydrates 6.3g	**2%**
Dietary Fiber 0.6g	**2%**
Sugars 3.1g	
Protein 6.1g	

Vitamin A 13%	•	Vitamin C 3%
Calcium 9%	•	Iron 4%

Nutrition Grade C
* Based on a 2000 calorie diet

Thyme chicken

Serves: 2
Time: 20 minutes
Ingredients:
- ½ lb. chicken tights, boneless and skinless
- 2 tablespoon olive oil, divided
- 2 garlic cloves, minced
- 2 teaspoons dried thyme
- ¼ cup sliced mushrooms
- Freshly ground salt and pepper
- 1 teaspoon lemon zest

Directions:
1. Season chicken tights with salt and pepper and lemon zest. Set aside for 20 minutes.
2. Heat large skillet over medium high heat and add olive oil.
3. Place chicken meat and cook for 7-10 minutes and cook until golden. Remove from the heat.
4. In another small skillet heat remaining oil and add garlic, thyme and mushrooms.
5. Cook for 5-7 minutes or until mushrooms are golden.
6. Pour mushrooms over chicken and stir well to combine.
7. Serve immediately.

Nutrition Facts

Serving Size 280 g

Amount Per Serving

Calories 540   Calories from Fat 208

	% Daily Value*
Total Fat 23.1g	**35%**
Saturated Fat 2.0g	**10%**
Trans Fat 0.0g	
Cholesterol 214mg	**71%**
Sodium 290mg	**12%**
Potassium 685mg	**20%**
Total Carbohydrates 2.1g	**1%**
Dietary Fiber 0.6g	**2%**
Protein 80.9g	

Vitamin A 1%	•	Vitamin C 5%
Calcium 6%	•	Iron 27%

Nutrition Grade B+
* Based on a 2000 calorie diet

Sausage-cauliflower casserole

Serves: 4
Time: 35 minutes
Ingredients:

- 1 tablespoon olive oil
- 1 cauliflower, cut into florets
- 1 ½ cups tomato sauce
- 2 oz. sliced pork sausages
- 1 cup mozzarella cheese, shredded
- ¼ teaspoon cayenne pepper
- Freshly ground salt and pepper

Directions:

1. Preheat oven to 400F and line baking tray with parchment paper.
2. Place cauliflower florets and drizzle with oil. Season with salt and pepper.
3. Bake cauliflower for 20-25 minutes and remove from the oven.
4. Place cauliflower in casserole dish and pour over tomato sauce.
5. Sprinkle with basil and add sliced sausages.
6. Top with mozzarella cheese and bake in oven at 350F until cheese melts.
7. Serve while still warm.

Nutrition Facts

Serving Size 138 g

Amount Per Serving

Calories 180	Calories from Fat 114

	% Daily Value*
Total Fat 12.7g	**20%**
Saturated Fat 4.8g	**24%**
Trans Fat 0.0g	
Cholesterol 27mg	**9%**
Sodium 758mg	**32%**
Potassium 348mg	**10%**
Total Carbohydrates 6.0g	**2%**
Dietary Fiber 1.4g	**6%**
Sugars 3.9g	
Protein 12.0g	

Vitamin A 11%	•	Vitamin C 11%
Calcium 21%	•	Iron 6%

Nutrition Grade B
* Based on a 2000 calorie diet

Grilled zucchinis with parmesan

Serves: 2
Time: 30 minutes
Ingredients:

- 2 medium zucchinis, cut lengthwise into ½-inch slices
- ¼ cup balsamic vinegar
- 2 tablespoons shredded parmesan
- Freshly ground pepper and salt
- 1 teaspoon garlic powder
- 1 tablespoon olive oil

Directions:

1. Preheat grill to 350F.
2. Place zucchinis in shallow dish and season with salt and pepper.
3. In a small bowl combine garlic powder, olive oil and vinegar.
4. Pour over zucchinis and set in refrigerate for 25 minutes.
5. Place zucchinis on the grill and cook for 5 minutes and flip in the other side.
6. Transfer to the plate and sprinkle with shredded parmesan.
7. Serve immediately.

Nutrition Facts

Serving Size 235 g

Amount Per Serving

Calories 102	Calories from Fat 66

% Daily Value*

Total Fat 7.4g	**11%**
Saturated Fat 1.1g	**5%**
Trans Fat 0.0g	
Cholesterol 0mg	**0%**
Sodium 21mg	**1%**
Potassium 551mg	**16%**
Total Carbohydrates 7.9g	**3%**
Dietary Fiber 2.3g	**9%**
Sugars 3.9g	
Protein 2.6g	

Vitamin A 8%	Vitamin C 56%
Calcium 3%	Iron 4%

Nutrition Grade A
* Based on a 2000 calorie diet

Squash and coconut slow-cooker curry

Serves: 4
Time: 6 hours
Ingredients:

- ½ cup onion, diced
- 1 garlic clove, minced
- 1 tomato, diced
- 1 ½ cup water
- 7 oz. coconut milk
- ¾ cup peas
- 1 ½ tablespoon mild curry
- ¾ cup black soy beans, soaked in water for 24 hours
- 1 ¼ cup butternut squash, peeled and cubed into 1-inch cubes
- ½ cup chopped kale
- ½ teaspoon salt
- 1 tablespoon chopped cilantro

Directions:

1. Add all ingredients in slow cooker, except kale and peas.
2. Stir well, cover and cook on high for 6 hours.
3. Around 30 minutes before serving add in the fresh peas and kale.
4. Give it a stir and continue cooking for those 30 minutes.
5. Serve while still hot with some brown rice and garnished with cilantro.

Nutrition Facts

Serving Size 249 g

Amount Per Serving

Calories 170	Calories from Fat 108
	% Daily Value*
Total Fat 12.0g	**18%**
Saturated Fat 10.5g	**53%**
Trans Fat 0.0g	
Cholesterol 0mg	**0%**
Sodium 309mg	**13%**
Potassium 455mg	**13%**
Total Carbohydrates 14.9g	**5%**
Dietary Fiber 4.0g	**16%**
Sugars 5.2g	
Protein 3.7g	

Vitamin A 126%	•	Vitamin C 58%
Calcium 6%	•	Iron 10%

Nutrition Grade A-
* Based on a 2000 calorie diet

Turkey-broccoli salad

Serves: 2
Time: 15 minutes
Ingredients:

- 1 tablespoon white vinegar
- 1 tablespoon olive oil
- Small pinch of salt
- ½ pound turkey breasts, cooked and shredded
- 6 oz. broccoli, shredded
- Freshly ground pepper
- 1 carrot, shredded

Directions:

1. In a small jar combine olive oil, salt, pepper and vinegar and cover.
2. Shake well and set aside.
3. In a large bowl combine shredded turkey, carrot and broccoli.
4. Pour over prepared dressing and toss to combine. Refrigerate for 30 minutes.
5. Serve after chilling in small bowls.

Nutrition Facts

Serving Size 244 g

Amount Per Serving

Calories 221	Calories from Fat 82
	% Daily Value*
Total Fat 9.2g	**14%**
Saturated Fat 1.4g	**7%**
Trans Fat 0.0g	
Cholesterol 49mg	**16%**
Sodium 1200mg	**50%**
Potassium 715mg	**20%**
Total Carbohydrates 13.5g	**5%**
Dietary Fiber 3.5g	**14%**
Sugars 7.0g	
Protein 22.0g	

Vitamin A 113%	•	Vitamin C 140%
Calcium 6%	•	Iron 13%

Nutrition Grade A
* Based on a 2000 calorie diet

Oven baked cauliflower steaks

Serves: 4
Time: 45 minutes
Ingredients:
- 1 head cauliflower, cut into steaks
- 1 tablespoon olive oil
- Freshly ground salt and pepper
- 1 teaspoon fennel seeds

Directions:
1. Preheat oven to 420F and line baking tray with parchment paper.
2. Place cauliflower steaks on baking sheet and brush with oil. Season with salt and pepper and sprinkle with fennel seeds.
3. Bake for 35-40 minutes or until cabbage is tender and edges are golden.
4. Serve when cooled slightly.

Nutrition Facts

Serving Size 71 g

Amount Per Serving

Calories 48	Calories from Fat 33

	% Daily Value*
Total Fat 3.6g	6%
Saturated Fat 0.5g	3%
Cholesterol 0mg	0%
Sodium 20mg	1%
Potassium 209mg	6%
Total Carbohydrates 3.8g	1%
Dietary Fiber 1.9g	7%
Sugars 1.6g	
Protein 1.4g	

Vitamin A 0%	•	Vitamin C 51%
Calcium 2%	•	Iron 2%

Nutrition Grade A-
* Based on a 2000 calorie diet

Lemon soup

Serves: 4
Time: 20 minutes
Ingredients:
- 30 oz. chicken stock, homemade
- ½ lemon juice
- ½ cup cauliflower, processed to resemble rice
- 2 springs dill, chopped
- 2 teaspoons chopped parsley
- 1 egg, whisked

Directions:
1. In a large sauce pan combine stock and cauliflower "rice".
2. Bring to boil over medium-high heat and reduce heat after to medium-low.
3. Simmer for 10minutes or until cauliflower is tender.
4. Gradually add whisked egg, stirring to create shreds.
5. Stir in lemon juice, parsley and stir well.
6. Remove from the heat and add dill. Stir once again and serve while still warm.

Nutrition Facts

Serving Size 237 g

Amount Per Serving

Calories 28	Calories from Fat 14
	% Daily Value*
Total Fat 1.6g	**2%**
Cholesterol 41mg	**14%**
Sodium 685mg	**29%**
Potassium 69mg	**2%**
Total Carbohydrates 1.4g	**0%**
Sugars 1.0g	
Protein 2.2g	

Vitamin A 2%	•	Vitamin C 11%
Calcium 2%	•	Iron 2%

Nutrition Grade A-
* Based on a 2000 calorie diet

Turkey meatballs

Serves: 4
Time: 15 minutes
Ingredients:
- 1 lb. ground turkey
- 1 egg
- ¼ cup chopped onion
- 2 garlic cloves, minced
- ½ teaspoon salt
- 3 basil leaves, chopped
- 2 teaspoons olive oil

Directions:
1. In a large bowl combine shopped basil, turkey meat, onion, garlic, egg and salt.
2. Mix well with hands and form meatballs.
3. Heat olive oil in large skillet over medium-high heat.
4. Cook meatballs until browned from all sides, or for 5-7 minutes.
5. Serve with some fresh salad.

Nutrition Facts

Serving Size 137 g

Amount Per Serving

Calories 262	Calories from Fat 143

	% Daily Value*
Total Fat 15.9g	**24%**
Saturated Fat 2.7g	**14%**
Cholesterol 157mg	**52%**
Sodium 428mg	**18%**
Potassium 339mg	**10%**
Total Carbohydrates 1.3g	**0%**
Protein 32.6g	

Vitamin A 1%	•	Vitamin C 2%
Calcium 4%	•	Iron 14%

Nutrition Grade B-
* Based on a 2000 calorie diet

Salmon cakes

Serves: 4
Time: 20 minutes
Ingredients:
- 6 oz. canned pink salmon
- 4 egg whites
- ½ cup almond meal
- 2 tablespoons pumpkin seeds, ground
- Small pinch of pepper
- 1 tablespoon olive oil

Directions:
1. In a large bowl combine egg whites, almond meal, pumpkin seeds and pepper.
2. Add drained salmon and stir well until combined.
3. Form 4 cakes from the mixture and set aside.
4. Heat olive oil in large non-stick skillet and add salmon cakes.
5. Cook for 5-7 minutes or until golden.
6. Transfer to the plate and serve.

Nutrition Facts

Serving Size 95 g

Amount Per Serving

Calories 195	Calories from Fat 127

% Daily Value*

Total Fat 14.1g	**22%**
Saturated Fat 1.7g	**9%**
Trans Fat 0.0g	
Cholesterol 19mg	**6%**
Sodium 53mg	**2%**
Potassium 339mg	**10%**
Total Carbohydrates 3.6g	**1%**
Dietary Fiber 1.7g	**7%**
Sugars 0.8g	
Protein 15.4g	

Vitamin A 1%	•	Vitamin C 0%
Calcium 5%	•	Iron 8%

Nutrition Grade B
* Based on a 2000 calorie diet

Dinner recipes

Feta cheese burgers

Serves: 4
Time: 15 minutes
Ingredients:

- 10 oz. minced beef
- 3 oz. feta cheese, crumbled
- 2 teaspoons dried parsley
- 1 teaspoon dried basil
- 1 oz. thick yogurt
- 1 teaspoon garlic powder
- Some olive oil – for frying

Directions:

1. Place all ingredients in a large bowl.
2. Stir well with metal spoon or mix with hands, until well combined.
3. Form patties from the mixture and heat olive oil in large non-stick skillet.
4. Fry patties for 5-7 minutes or until browned,
5. Serve immediately.

Nutrition Facts

Serving Size 94 g

Amount Per Serving

Calories 190	Calories from Fat 81
	% Daily Value*
Total Fat 8.9g	**14%**
Saturated Fat 4.8g	**24%**
Cholesterol 82mg	**27%**
Sodium 284mg	**12%**
Potassium 310mg	**9%**
Total Carbohydrates 1.4g	**0%**
Sugars 1.1g	
Protein 24.7g	

Vitamin A 3%	•	Vitamin C 2%
Calcium 11%	•	Iron 75%

Nutrition Grade B
* Based on a 2000 calorie diet

Green beans and pine nuts

Serves: 4
Time: 15 minutes
Ingredients:
- 1 lb. green beans, cut into ½.inch pieces
- ¼ cup pine nuts
- 2 teaspoons olive oil
- 1 tablespoon lime juice

Directions:
1. Cook beans in large pot of salted water for 5 minutes and drain well.
2. Meanwhile heat olive oil in large skillet and add pine nuts. Toast them for couple minutes and add cooked green beans.
3. Stir well and transfer to the bowl.
4. Pour over oil from the skillet and drizzle with lemon juice.
5. Toss to combine and serve.

Nutrition Facts

Serving Size 124 g

Amount Per Serving

Calories 112	Calories from Fat 75

	% Daily Value*
Total Fat 8.3g	**13%**
Saturated Fat 0.8g	**4%**
Cholesterol 0mg	**0%**
Sodium 7mg	**0%**
Potassium 288mg	**8%**
Total Carbohydrates 9.2g	**3%**
Dietary Fiber 4.2g	**17%**
Sugars 1.9g	
Protein 3.2g	

Vitamin A 16%	•	Vitamin C 31%	
Calcium 4%	•	Iron 9%	

Nutrition Grade A
* Based on a 2000 calorie diet

Cauliflower rice with zucchinis

Serves: 2
Time:
Ingredients:

- 2 cups cauliflower "rice" (simply process cauliflower to get 2 cups), steamed
- 1 medium zucchini, cut into ½-inch cubes
- ½ teaspoon chili powder
- ¼ teaspoon ground cumin
- Freshly ground salt and pepper
- ½ tablespoon lemon juice
- 2 tablespoons chopped mint
- 1 small onion, chopped
- 2 garlic cloves, minced
- Some olive oil – for frying

Directions:

1. Heat large non-stick skillet over medium heat. Add olive oil and when heated add onion. Cook for 5 minutes or until tender.
2. Add garlic and cook for 30 seconds.
3. Add zucchinis; cook for 5 minutes, or until just tender.
4. Reduce heat to low and stir in the spices; season with salt and pepper, to taste.
5. Add steamed cauliflower "rice" and toss to combine well.
6. Set aside for 5 minutes before serving.

Nutrition Facts

Serving Size 246 g

Amount Per Serving

Calories 63	Calories from Fat 4

	% Daily Value*
Total Fat 0.4g	**1%**
Cholesterol 0mg	**0%**
Sodium 44mg	**2%**
Potassium 654mg	**19%**
Total Carbohydrates 13.4g	**4%**
Dietary Fiber 4.8g	**19%**
Sugars 5.7g	
Protein 4.0g	

Vitamin A 9%	•	Vitamin C 115%
Calcium 6%	•	Iron 9%

Nutrition Grade A
* Based on a 2000 calorie diet

Soy beans salad with asparagus and dill

Serves: 2
Time: 10 minutes
Ingredients:

- ½ cup can black soy beans, rinsed, drained
- 1 garlic clove, minced
- ¼ cup diced tomatoes
- ½ cup diced asparagus
- 2 tablespoons lemon juice
- 1 tablespoon fresh dill, chopped
- 1 tablespoon olive oil
- Freshly ground salt

Directions:

1. Place asparagus in a large pot and cover with water. Simmer for 2 minutes or until crisp-tender. Drain and place in a large bowl.
2. Add soy beans, tomato, dill and drizzle over with olive oil and lemon juice.
3. Season with freshly ground salt and toss to combine. Serve in a small bowls

Nutrition Facts

Serving Size 147 g

Amount Per Serving

Calories 161	Calories from Fat 97
	% Daily Value*
Total Fat 10.8g	**17%**
Saturated Fat 1.6g	**8%**
Cholesterol 0mg	**0%**
Sodium 203mg	**8%**
Potassium 197mg	**6%**
Total Carbohydrates 10.4g	**3%**
Dietary Fiber 7.3g	**29%**
Sugars 2.6g	
Protein 8.0g	

Vitamin A 12%	•	Vitamin C 22%
Calcium 8%	•	Iron 19%

Nutrition Grade B
* Based on a 2000 calorie diet

Roasted tuna with grapefruit

Serves: 2
Time: 20 minutes
Ingredients:

- 2 5 oz. tuna steaks
- 1 tablespoon olive oil
- ½ white grapefruit
- 1 tablespoon minced shallots
- Freshly ground salt

Directions:

1. Preheat oven to 475F.
2. Grate 1 teaspoon grapefruit peel and reserve.
3. Cut off remaining peel and slice grapefruit in 6 slices; remove the seeds.
4. Combine shallots and grapefruit zest in a bowl.
5. Drizzle with olive oil and season with salt.
6. Spread the mixture over baking tray and top with tuna steaks.
7. Roast for 5 minutes and remove from the oven. Top with grapefruit slices and bake for 5 minutes more.
8. Serve while still hot.

Nutrition Facts

Serving Size 186 g

Amount Per Serving

Calories 335	Calories from Fat 143
	% Daily Value*
Total Fat 15.9g	**25%**
Saturated Fat 3.3g	**16%**
Cholesterol 69mg	**23%**
Sodium 71mg	**3%**
Potassium 519mg	**15%**
Total Carbohydrates 3.4g	**1%**
Sugars 2.2g	
Protein 42.7g	

Vitamin A 79%	•	Vitamin C 19%
Calcium 2%	•	Iron 11%

Nutrition Grade A-
* Based on a 2000 calorie diet

Soy bean and spinach slow-cooker enchiladas

Serves: 8
Time: 3 hours
Ingredients:

- 10 oz. chopped spinach
- 15 oz. soy beans, cooked rinsed and drained
- ½ teaspoon ground cumin
- 6 cups chopped lettuce
- ½ cup grape tomatoes, halved
- ½ cucumber, halved and sliced
- 3 tablespoons lime juice, fresh
- 3 cups salsa
- 8 almond flour tortillas
- ½ cup cashew halves - -processed in food blender for 15 seconds

Directions:

1. In a medium bowl mash half of the soy beans. Add cumin, spinach, ¼ cup processed cashews, remaining soy beans, salt and pepper; stir to combine.
2. Spread 1 cup salsa in the bottom of 4 quart slow cooker.
3. Divide bean mixture evenly between almond flour tortillas and place them seam side down on top of salsa and pour over remaining salsa and cashews.
4. Cover and cook on low for 3 hours.
5. Combine lettuce, lime juice, salt and pepper in a bowl; toss to combine.
6. Serve whit prepared enchiladas.

Nutrition Facts

Serving Size 266 g

Amount Per Serving

Calories 95	Calories from Fat 40

% Daily Value*

Total Fat 4.4g	**7%**
Saturated Fat 0.8g	**4%**
Trans Fat 0.0g	
Cholesterol 0mg	**0%**
Sodium 619mg	**26%**
Potassium 651mg	**19%**
Total Carbohydrates 12.6g	**4%**
Dietary Fiber 3.1g	**12%**
Sugars 4.6g	
Protein 4.2g	

Vitamin A 75%	Vitamin C 26%
Calcium 7%	Iron 18%

Nutrition Grade A
* Based on a 2000 calorie diet

Snacks

"Hummus" and veggies

Serves: 4
Time: 20 minutes
Ingredients:

- ½ cup fresh lemon juice
- 4 cups zucchini, peeled grated
- ¼ cup olive oil
- ½ garlic clove, crushed
- ½ teaspoon ground cumin
- ¼ teaspoon salt
- ¾ cup tahini
- 1/8 teaspoon cayenne pepper
- Vegetables by your choice – celery, carrot sticks

Directions:

1. Place garlic in food processor and add the zucchinis, lemon juice, spices and sesame paste.
2. Process until smooth; add water if needed to thin.
3. Serve with vegetables by your choice.

Nutrition Facts

Serving Size 203 g

Amount Per Serving

Calories 403	Calories from Fat 336

	% Daily Value*
Total Fat 37.3g	**57%**
Saturated Fat 5.5g	**27%**
Cholesterol 0mg	**0%**
Sodium 217mg	**9%**
Potassium 528mg	**15%**
Total Carbohydrates 14.2g	**5%**
Dietary Fiber 5.6g	**22%**
Sugars 2.8g	
Protein 9.3g	

Vitamin A 6%	•	Vitamin C 56%
Calcium 21%	•	Iron 26%

Nutrition Grade B
* Based on a 2000 calorie diet

"Tortilla Chips"

Serves: 4
Time: 30 minutes
Ingredients:

- ½ cup coconut flour
- ½ cup almond meal
- ½ tablespoon lime juice
- ½ cup warm water
- ½ teaspoon salt
- 1/8 teaspoon chili powder
- ¼ teaspoon cumin

Directions:

1. Combine all ingredients in a bowl and stir until ball forms.
2. Let the dough rest for 15 minutes and meanwhile preheat the oven to 400F.
3. Transfer the dough onto ungreased baking sheet and press with hands to making it thin as possible.
4. Cut with sharp knife into desired form and bake for 20 minutes.
5. Serve when cooled.

Nutrition Facts

Serving Size 52 g

Amount Per Serving

Calories 105	Calories from Fat 84

	% Daily Value*
Total Fat 9.3g	**14%**
Saturated Fat 3.4g	**17%**
Trans Fat 0.0g	
Cholesterol 0mg	**0%**
Sodium 295mg	**12%**
Potassium 127mg	**4%**
Total Carbohydrates 4.2g	**1%**
Dietary Fiber 2.4g	**10%**
Sugars 1.1g	
Protein 2.9g	

Vitamin A 1%	•	Vitamin C 1%
Calcium 3%	•	Iron 11%

Nutrition Grade B+
* Based on a 2000 calorie diet

Pumpkin bars

Serves: 4
Time: 45 minutes
Ingredients:

- ½ cup cooked pumpkin cubes
- ½ medium banana
- ½ teaspoon pumpkin pie spice
- ½ tablespoon ground flaxseed meal
- 2 tablespoons chopped walnuts
- 1 tablespoon chopped dried cranberries
- ½ cup almond meal
- ¼ teaspoon grated orange zest

Directions:

1. Preheat oven to 350F and line baking pan 4x2 inch with parchment paper.
2. Place pumpkin, banana, almond meal, cranberries, orange zest, pumpkin spice and ground flaxseeds meal in food processor. Pulse until smooth.
3. Stir in walnuts and transfer the mixture into prepared baking pan.
4. Smooth the mixture top with spatula and bake in preheated oven for 40 minutes or until top is golden.
5. Set on wire rack to cool and slice into 8 bars.
6. Keep in airtight container wrapped in parchment paper.

Nutrition Facts

Serving Size 47 g

Amount Per Serving

Calories 112	Calories from Fat 75
	% Daily Value*
Total Fat 8.3g	**13%**
Saturated Fat 0.6g	**3%**
Trans Fat 0.0g	
Cholesterol 0mg	**0%**
Sodium 1mg	**0%**
Potassium 214mg	**6%**
Total Carbohydrates 7.6g	**3%**
Dietary Fiber 2.3g	**9%**
Sugars 2.6g	
Protein 3.8g	

Vitamin A 22%	*	Vitamin C 6%
Calcium 4%	*	Iron 4%

Nutrition Grade A
* Based on a 2000 calorie diet

Raw banana sandwiches

Serves: 4
Time: 5 minutes
Ingredients:
- ¼ cup almond butter
- 2 apples
- ¼ teaspoon cinnamon
- 1 tablespoon pumpkin puree
- 1/8 teaspoon vanilla, pure
- 1/8 teaspoon pumpkin pie spice

Directions:
1. Prepare the butter; place almond butter, pumpkin and spices in food processor; pulse until combined and creamy.
2. Slice the apples into thin rounds.
3. Top each slice with 1 teaspoon prepared butter and sandwich with other apple slice.
4. Sprinkle additionally with cinnamon and serve.

Nutrition Facts

Serving Size 106 g

Amount Per Serving

Calories 150	Calories from Fat 105

	% Daily Value*
Total Fat 11.7g	**18%**
Saturated Fat 7.3g	**36%**
Trans Fat 0.0g	
Cholesterol 31mg	**10%**
Sodium 83mg	**3%**
Potassium 102mg	**3%**
Total Carbohydrates 12.7g	**4%**
Dietary Fiber 2.3g	**9%**
Sugars 9.5g	
Protein 0.4g	

Vitamin A 7%	Vitamin C 12%
Calcium 1%	Iron 2%

Nutrition Grade D
* Based on a 2000 calorie diet

Aromatic almonds

Serves: 4
Time: 70 minutes
Ingredients:

- 1 cup whole almonds
- ¼ teaspoon cinnamon
- ½ tablespoon orange peel powder
- 1/8 teaspoon nutmeg
- 1/8 teaspoon salt
- ¼ tablespoon coconut oil

Directions:

1. Preheat oven to 250F and line baking tray with parchment paper.
2. Place almond in a large bowl and drizzle with coconut oil; toss to coat.
3. Add spices and shake until coated evenly.
4. Arrange almonds onto baking sheet in single layer and place in the oven.
5. Bake for 1 hour, stirring occasionally.
6. Serve when cooled or still slightly warm.

Nutrition Facts

Serving Size 25 g

Amount Per Serving

Calories 145	Calories from Fat 115

	% Daily Value*
Total Fat 12.8g	**20%**
Saturated Fat 1.7g	**8%**
Trans Fat 0.0g	
Cholesterol 0mg	**0%**
Sodium 74mg	**3%**
Potassium 175mg	**5%**
Total Carbohydrates 5.2g	**2%**
Dietary Fiber 3.0g	**12%**
Sugars 1.0g	
Protein 5.0g	

Vitamin A 0%	•	Vitamin C 0%
Calcium 7%	•	Iron 5%

Nutrition Grade B+
* Based on a 2000 calorie diet

Yummy snack

Serves: 20 balls
Time: 35 minutes
Ingredients:

- 1 cup mashed bananas
- 1 cup finely grated apple
- 1 ½ cup almond meal
- ¾ cup frozen raspberries
- ½ cup dried cranberries
- 1 teaspoon ground cinnamon
- Small pinch salt
- ½ cup walnuts, chopped

Directions:

1. Combine mashed bananas and apple in a bowl.
2. Add almond meal and stir to combine.
3. Add cranberries, cinnamon, walnuts and salt; mix well.
4. Add the raspberries and stir until combined.
5. Preheat oven to 350F and line baking tray with parchment paper.
6. Spoon around soup spoon of the mixture and roll to form ball. Place onto baking sheet and bake in preheated oven for 20 minutes.
7. Set on wire rack to cool and serve.
8. Keep in airtight container.

Nutrition Facts

Serving Size 46 g

Amount Per Serving

Calories 40   Calories from Fat 17

	% Daily Value*
Total Fat 1.9g	**3%**
Trans Fat 0.0g	
Cholesterol 0mg	**0%**
Sodium 1mg	**0%**
Potassium 65mg	**2%**
Total Carbohydrates 5.6g	**2%**
Dietary Fiber 1.1g	**4%**
Sugars 3.7g	
Protein 0.9g	

Vitamin A 0%	•	Vitamin C 6%
Calcium 1%	•	Iron 1%

Nutrition Grade A-
* Based on a 2000 calorie diet

Final Thoughts

Nutrition and fitness experts from *WebMD* highly recommend you plan your day to lose weight. This is exactly what this Ketogenic Diet does for you. Change is tough and quite frankly reducing your carbs and boosting fats is going to be a shock to your system initially. A good one but still a shock nonetheless.

*If you commit your heart and soul to the Ketogenic Diet Rapid Weight Loss Plan you WILL lose up to a pound a day, or 30 pounds in thirty days, but ONLY if you commit!

You will not lose weight and make it stick if you don't have a plan, both short term and long term.

It really helps to have your meals planned and healthy low-carb, high-fat, and moderate protein snacks handy in a pinch. Your willpower is weak when your energy levels dip or you are just plain hungry.

Make the time to set out your exercise and eating plan at least the day before, and preferably a week in advance. This is going to increase your success rate. Take the sample meal ideas from this guide and build off them. Use the underlying fast weight loss eating strategy you have learned with this book to develop your fat blasting plan farther.

Losing fat is hard work and by switching up your typical balance of energy burn with the Ketogenic Diet, studies show you can lose up to 30 pounds in the first month! That's got to make you smile!

Make the time to understand the mechanics of this quick weight loss diet, commit to regular and effective high intensity interval training, and you **WILL** get skinny **FAST**! I'm not about to argue with science and neither should you.

It's time for you to make the changes you need to get healthy and happy in your skin. Now you've got the tools to reach your fat loss goals quickly and make them stick. Say **YES** and get started today. Promise you'll be happy you did!

Thank you for downloading this book!

I hope this book helps you jumpstart your fat loss journey. If you enjoyed this book, then I'd like to ask you for a favor, would you be kind enough to leave a review for this book by clicking here. It'd be greatly appreciated!

Thank you and good luck!

Henry Brooke

Check Out My Other Books

Below you'll find some of my other popular books that are popular on Amazon and Kindle as well. Simply click on the links below to check them out. Alternatively, you can visit my author page on Amazon to see other work done by me.

The Autoimmune Eating Guide: A Paleo Approach To Reversing Autoimmune Symptoms

Low Carb Diet Guide: The Ultimate 7 Day Guide to Jump-Start Fat Loss Fast and Start Feeling Great Today

Essential Oils Allergy Cure: The Definitive Guide On Using Essential Oils To Completely Eliminate Seasonal Allergy Symptoms

Get Your Free eBook Here

Click Here To Download Your Free eBook "Extreme Weight Loss Secrets: How To Lose 20 Pounds In 3 Weeks"